I0440052

Simply Weight Loss

By Dr. Mike Cockrell

Laurel Rose Publishing
laurelrosepublishing@gmail.com

Dedication

I would like to thank my wife, Lisa, for all of the support she has been for me throughout my career. Her insight and inspiration is unending. Thanks baby. I love you.

I would also like to thank the hundreds and hundreds of patients who have trusted me with their health and well-being. They are the ones that allow me to continue to hone the weight loss program and see the results of their efforts. The changes in their lives are phenomenal.

I would like to thank my clinic staff at Cockrell Family Medical Center for all of the long hours of dedicated effort they put forth in making sure that our clinic operates at peak performance.

I would like to thank my friends, family members and especially my children who inspire me to reach above and beyond my limits each and every day of my life.

The key to great success is to surround yourself with other people who are always challenging you to be better tomorrow than you were today.

Finally, I would like to offer a special thanks to Chad Martin for all of his support in making this project a reality. His willingness to forge the path and then leave a trail for others to follow is greatly appreciated.

Table of Contents

Simply Weight Loss

Why we struggle with our weight...

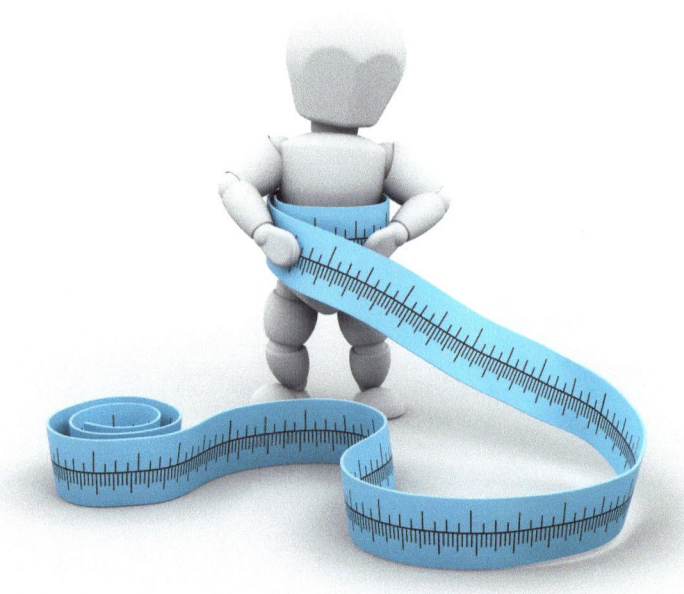

As a practicing family physician, weight loss is likely one of the biggest health related issues that I deal with each and every day in my clinical practice. Not only do I see this as a major issue for my patient's but I too have struggled with weight issues. That struggle, combined with my desire to help teach others how to have weight loss success in their lives, has led me to write this book.

For most of us, it is not enough to be told you need to do this or that. We really seem to have more success when we understand the basic principles of why we need to do the task.

I have found that in dealing with people from all different backgrounds that we do better when we know the *"WHY"* behind the process. That is why we are going to start with the basics. I am going to share this information with you in the same way that I share it with my patients in the clinic.

My goal at the end of this process is that you will not only have a plan that is as individual as you are, but that you will understand the impact that the excess weight has on you physically, emotionally and mentally.

If we can understand our "*WHY*", then you truly can make the changes that are necessary to get your weight under control but more importantly, you will be able to take control of all areas of your life.

Everyone knows that being overweight is bad. We know the physical, psychological, emotional and financial devastation it can cause. We also know that losing just 10 pounds of excess weight can have a profound effect on how we feel and how we act. It affects how we feel in so many ways not to mention the positive effects on your blood pressure and your blood sugar.

These small changes are just enough for many people to eliminate daily medications that have the potential for significant side effects.

The true essence of success in our lives is to be able to live life to the fullest each and every day and do it in a way that seems natural to us. If you find that you are having to force your way through each and every day or through each and every step of this program, you will FAIL, not only in reaching your weight loss goals but also in every other aspect of your life. *I refuse to allow that to happen.*

Even though I don't know you personally, my goal is to write this book in a manner that you feel like it is written with only you in mind. I want this book to resonate with you as if I were sitting right next to you in my office sharing the hows and whys of weight loss with you directly.

So, in order for us to do that, we need to roll up our sleeves and start this whole process from the beginning.

- **We** will look at what we have been doing for the past 10, 20, 30, or more years that have actually landed at this place in time.

- **We** will work through the science behind the madness so that we have a good understanding of what has gone wrong.

- **We** will create a plan of action that will help you get to the goals you desire to achieve.

TOGETHER, we will simply learn how to cut the weight and keep it off.

So let's dig in and get started!

Why Do I Keep Gaining Weight?

This is likely the most common question that I deal with every day. People are always asking, "***Why do I keep gaining weight, no matter what I do?***"

In order to fully understand what we need to do to correct your weight gain, it is essential to understand some of the science behind how you have gotten here.

I know, I know; you hate science and why don't you just cut to the chase and give me a plan to shed the pounds.

We will get to that, but you ***have*** to understand that if there were one single plan that would cut the weight off of you, we would not be having this conversation in the first place. We would all do the plan and we would all be skinny. Well, look around. I don't think anyone has actually found that plan.

Anyone can drop 5, 10 or 15 pounds in the short term.

In fact, most of the people I deal with can shed 10 pounds in the first 2 to 3 weeks of being on their program. The key is not in being able to lose the weight. ***True success comes from being able to keep the weight off once you reach your goal.***

Have you ever experienced this yo-yo phenomenon that goes along with weight loss?

Do you know anyone else that has?

I bet you have and I bet you know a dozen or more close friends that have had the same up and down experience. What good is it to lose the weight if 2 months later it is all right back or, worse yet, you are heavier than before?

If we want to stop the yo-yo weight rollercoaster, we have to understand **why** we do that and then we have to structure our program to prevent that process from ever occurring again.

The problem is that this phenomenon is multi-faceted. That is, there are a ton of different reasons and a lot of physiology that is involved in why we cycle this way.

That's right. Until you understand some of the basics of what causes this, you will struggle with keeping the weight off. Therefore, we are going to start by trying to explain how this whole system we call our body interacts with itself and the outside world.

As we gain a better understanding of what is happening on the inside, we can modify what we are doing on the outside to maximize out ability to lose weight and keep it off for the long haul.

One of the key premises that I work with in my practice is that we are very simply unique creatures. None of us are exactly the same and therefore we each may need a little different program to make things work. That is why I am convinced that there will never be a perfect diet because **one size will never fit us all**.

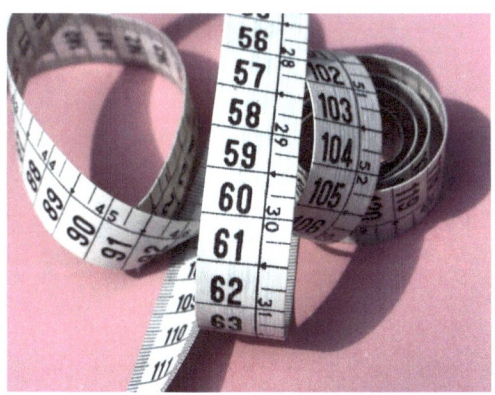

With that in mind, I find that if you understand the basics of what is going on in your body when you eat certain foods, then we can begin to identify the **Simple Things** that we need to modify in order to achieve our weight loss goals. This is going to take a little bit of work on your part, but anyone can do this.

How Food Affects Us

"Rich, fatty foods are like destiny; they too shape our ends."-- Author Unknown

Do you realize that food is a drug?

 That's right. Food can affect your body and your cellular physiology just like drugs can. With that in mind, why do we take the things we put in our mouths for granted?

Have you ever wondered what that honey bun was doing other than tickling your taste buds with its sweet deliciousness?

Alright, you caught me. I am a junk food junkie. I have been as far back as I can remember. The problem is that my body reacts in certain ways when I eat junk foods and that reaction is what keeps me coming back for more.

Do you have a particular food that you crave?

If so, that might not be a coincidence. Our bodies are affected differently by different foods and each one of us reacts differently to certain foods as well. Some of this may be coded at the genetic level and some of it is influenced by our environment.

Either way, we are not here to debate that issue, we are here to learn how to use this idea to our advantage to lose weight and keep it off.

If we want to have true long term success with our weight, we need to have at least a basic understanding of **how food affects us** and how we need to change the way we think about food.

There have been way too many "**fad**" diets in the past and these just seem to confuse the issue:

- Do I need low carb?

- Do I need low fat?

- What about protein, is it good or bad?

The honest truth is that **your body needs sugar, fat and proteins** in order to function optimally.

Any time you sacrifice one or more of these groups to follow a fad, you are likely creating failure. Don't get me wrong; you can lose weight with any of these programs. If you couldn't do you think there would be so many? The problem is that **we want to lose the weight and keep it off**. The keeping it off part is where most of these programs begin to break down. I have never met anyone that could sustain a low carb diet for long periods of time and be successful at keeping the weight off.

Any time you do this you are altering your physiology in an unnatural way and that is doomed to fail. What I want you to understand as we go through this process is how you are affected by different foods and how you can begin to manage your eating to optimize your natural physiology.

I know you are scratching your head saying "I can't do that." but I am going to teach you some very simple techniques that will allow you to see how foods are affecting you and then we are going to modify our habits so that we can achieve long-term success and **keep the weight off forever.**

As we begin to look at the different food groups, it is important to remember that not all sugars, fats and proteins are the same. That's right. We will be focusing on those foods that actually work with your body for long-term health benefits.

The simplest concept to understand is that **natural sugars obtained from fruits and vegetables are great for you.**

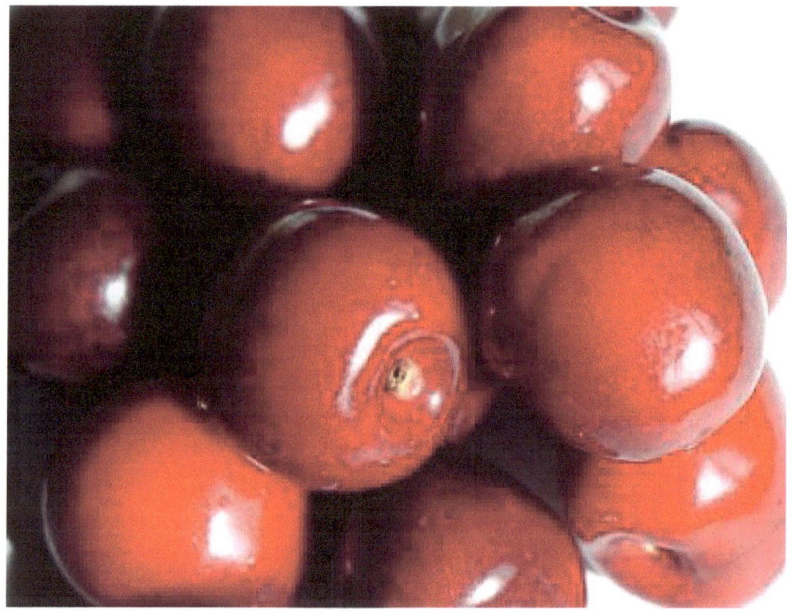

The processed sugars that are found in most processed foods and fast foods are of no benefit and in fact they work to wreck your system in a multitude of ways. I know, you thought you were going to get to eat anything you wanted without any personal responsibility. Not!

We also know that not all fats are created equally. We will discuss these in more detail but for now suffice it to say that **your fast food habit has got to be greatly curtailed**.

I believe that any of us can tolerate a bit of badness in our diets but the problem I see in my clinic is simply that most people have developed a fast food addiction that runs rampant. In order to gain control over our weight, we have to control these habits.

It is time to take charge of your destiny, your health and your likelihood of a long life.

The Science Behind The Madness

"You've got to say, I think that if I keep working at this and want it badly enough, I can have it. It's called perseverance."—Lee Iacocca

There have been some tremendous strides over the past 10 years in the area of weight loss. We have known for years about issues related to the basic hormones in our body. Things like thyroid and insulin have been taunted as significant contributors to weight gain.

The problem is that I hear people all the time talk about how their metabolism is slow and their thyroid is not working. We use these hormonal issues as excuses to keep us fat. ***I will not stand for that.***

If you do have a hormonal imbalance, ***you need to get it fixed***.

It is likely that the crap you have been eating for the past 20 years is actually the reason why your hormonal system is wrecked in the first place. Regardless of why it is there, you need to fix it and get slim.

In addition to thyroid and insulin, we now know that there are several other major players in the weight loss arena. Hormones such as **adiponectin** and **grehlin** have made their way into most of the literature about weight loss. It is possible, no, it is likely, that you have some type of imbalance in one or more of these systems.

There are some things that we can do to support these systems that we will get to but the main thing you need to do is begin to ***change the way you eat and many of these issues will fix themselves.***

Your body has a remarkable ability to heal itself.

If you will give it the basics it needs it will restore most of its major functions without special cocktails and potions. When you get rid of the foods that are hindering these systems and begin to provide your body with the *"super foods"* that can help restore your balance it is amazing what you get.

Understanding How Food Works

One of the main premises of this book is how to make weight loss simple.

 No matter where you look today you can find dozens and dozens of books about dieting and weight loss. ***Everybody has a system. Everybody has a plan.***

The problem that I have with most of those is just that. They have a plan and as long as you can follow a detailed, meal-to-meal plan you will lose weight.

Most of the people that I talk to in my practice about weight loss are not able to follow a rigid plan. They are busy trying to make it through their day; up in the morning, rushing to get out of the house to get to work. They try to eat around their work schedule then rush home, trying to prepare meals for everyone in the household.

There have been many of my patients that realize when they diet, the whole family diets. It is difficult to prepare a meal for the dieters in the family and something else for everyone else.

One of my primary goals in this program is to educate people about how food works in their body and how they can ***use that knowledge to lose the weight they need to lose.***

For many of you this section many seem redundant, but I feel that it is a necessary evil in order to have a good understanding of how the things we eat actually affect our weight, our hormonal systems and our physiological make up.

The more you understand the effects of food on your body the better you will be at making good decisions.

Let's face it. **No one** has been sitting on top of you for the last 10 or 20 years forcing you to eat the crap that has led you down this path of weight loss.

You have done that to yourself.

Much of it has been done simply because you do not really understand how food works and how it affects your body at the cellular level.

All of that is going to change over the next few minutes.

Breaking Through the Diet Myths

"Your goals, minus your doubts, equals your reality."—
Ralph Marston

As we try to understand more about how food works in our bodies, it is important to know that not all of the knowledge that is propagated in this world is correct. That's right.

If you are like most people you have probably been exposed to at least 10 to 20 fad diets over the years. Who has not heard of the **"low carb"** diet or the "**low fat**" diet or the **"high protein"** diet?

The fact is that if you want to be able to live your life and keep the weight off, *you need to understand the basics of how carbs, fats and proteins work in your body.* Education is essential to success.

The purpose of this section is to try to clear up some of the most common myths that are told about weight loss.

Myth #1:   Carbohydrates are bad and need to be avoided.

The fact is that all carbohydrates are **not** created equally.

The "low carb" model has been around for many years now and most if not all of us have tried the "low carb" approach at one time or another. The thing about "low carb" is that you can shed pounds using this approach, however, most of that weight is going to find its way back to you as soon as you stop the diet.

This poses 2 main problems.

First, you gain all of the weight back. Who wants to do that? When you started the diet did you say to yourself, "I'm going to lose this 10 pounds this week and then gain it back next month"? Not likely. We usually believe that if we can shed it fast that will be our jumpstart to even further success with losing weight. That usually does not work.

Second, this process usually sets you up for more yo-yo weight loss (and gain). Any time you severely restrict you intake of a specific group of foods, you are setting yourself up for ultimate failure. If we are going to lose weight and be able to keep that weight off of our bodies, we have to learn how to make friends with all of the foods our there.

Carbohydrates are not bad.

There are some forms of carbohydrates that I strongly recommend that you avoid most of the time but there has never been anyone who completely wrecked their weight loss by eating one candy bar. It doesn't happen. What happens is that we eat one then another then another until the entire bag is gone; *and therein lies the problem.*

Your body **needs** carbohydrates for energy. *In fact, most of us need as much as 50% of our calories to come from carbohydrates*. What we have to understand is that all carbs are not equal.

That means that you must understand how food works in order to be able to make friends with them.

One of the key issues to understand when it comes to carbohydrates is the relationship that eating carbs has with your body's production of insulin, *the key hormone in energy management*.

When you eat carbohydrates, your blood sugar levels rise causing your pancreas to secrete insulin. This release of insulin acts like a shuttle bus in your system. The insulin picks up the circulating blood sugar (glucose) and transports it to those muscles and other tissues that need the sugar for energy. This system is **essential** for energy management in our bodies.

In a normal individual, keeping a supply of blood sugar available throughout the day is essential to keeping your energy production and management optimal.

One of the reasons I believe that we see our weight increase year after year after year is due to this insulin issue.

Year after year of eating high glycemic carbohydrates and unhealthy processed sugars causes your insulin levels to rise. The more the insulin levels rise in your body the more efficient you become at storing this blood sugar and converting it to fat.

Let me explain in another way.

Insulin is like a dump truck in your system and blood sugar is like a gravel pit. As you eat food the gravel pit (glucose) gets filled up. When you have the right amount of dump trucks (insulin) hauling the gravel to different sites you maintain an optimal balance for energy management.

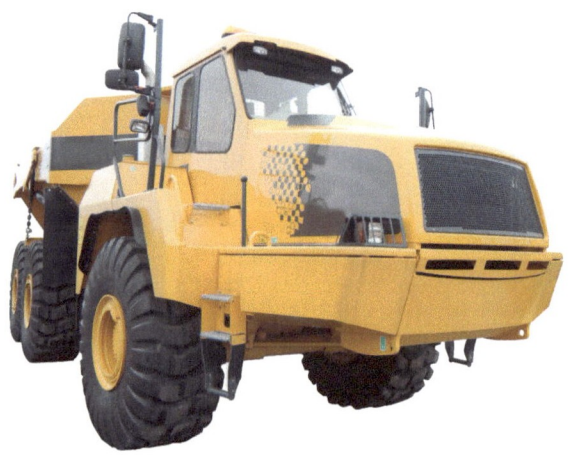

Over time, we continue to eat bad carbohydrates and our insulin levels continues to rise in our system. In essence, we are constantly adding new dump trucks (insulin) without really building a bigger gravel pit (glucose).

As we age, the carbohydrates that we eat get picked up more rapidly because we have all of these new dump trucks (insulin) and the muscles and tissue get over whelmed and can not use the gravel (blood sugar) when it gets delivered.

When this happens, the dump trucks need to be unloaded so they get directed to the closest storage facility (the liver) for unloading. *As the blood sugar gets dumped in the liver for storage it eventually gets converted to fat and stored around our waist lines and other areas.*

I know this analogy is silly but it helps to understand the mechanism. If you can understand the mechanism not matter how silly the analogy, you can then begin to make decisions that work in your favor instead of against you.

The key to managing the carbohydrate system is to make most of your carbohydrates natural. That is, they should come from fruits and vegetables not from a paper wrapper or a box.

Carbohydrates (starches and sugars) are by far the greatest stimulators of insulin. That is why *it is so important to eat more natural or low glycemic carbohydrates*. These sugars to do raise the insulin levels as high or as fast as the high glycemic carbohydrates (processed sugars, breads, cereals) do.

The Glycemic Index and What It Means

I realize at this point that I have just discussed low glycemic and high glycemic carbohydrates but I have not really given you the definition of these terms. Since I am trying to educate you on these topics, we should clarify these issues before moving forward.

The glycemic index (GI) was created in 1981 by Dr. David Jenkins and provides us with a way to determine which foods raise blood sugar the highest thereby stimulating insulin production and increasing weight gain.

Carbohydrates with a high blood sugar and insulin response score high on the GI scale and carb sources with a low blood sugar and insulin response score low on the GI scale.

If you'd actually like to find out the numerical value of a food's GI or GL, you may do so at www.GlycemicIndex.com. Here are some numbers to guide you:

Glycemic Index

 <55 – Low

55-70 – Moderate

>70 – High

Low Glycemic Foods Examples

Cereals, Breads, and Grains

Choose cereals that are based on barley, bran, or oats.

All-Bran (50), rolled oats (51), Natural Muesli (40), and Special K (54).

Low GI breads include whole wheat (49), sourdough (54), and pumpernickel (49).

Other low GI products are spaghetti (32), wheat tortillas (30), pearled barley (22).

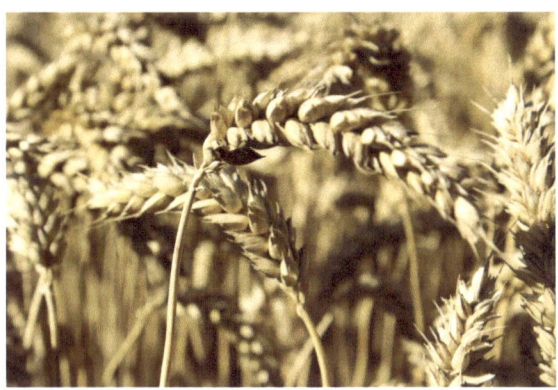

Fruits and Vegetables

Fruits and vegetables are an important part of any healthy diet, and many have a low GI.

Some good choices are green peas (30), raw carrots (16), broccoli (10), cauliflower (15), lettuce (10), green beans (15), yams (35), and cabbage (10).

Low GI fruits include peaches (28), apples (34), plums (24), cherries (22), oranges (40), strawberries (40), and grapefruit (25).

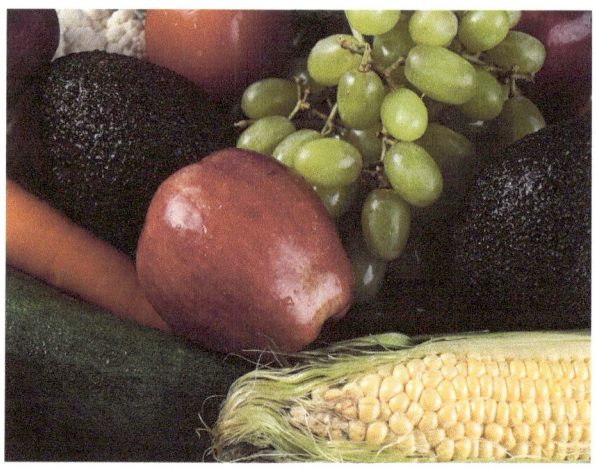

Dairy

Low-fat and nonfat dairy products can be a great source of calcium and protein.

Good dairy choices are skim milk (32), chocolate milk (42), and yogurt (33).

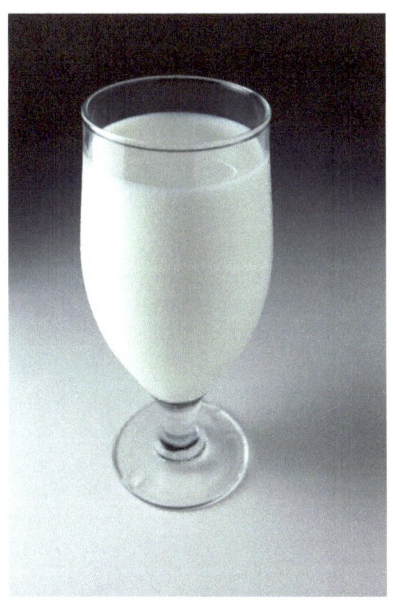

Legumes

Legumes are generally low in fat and packed with nutrients, fiber, and protein.

Some low GI legumes are red lentils (21), green lentils (30), pinto beans (45), split peas (32), kidney beans (52), chickpeas (42), and navy beans (31).

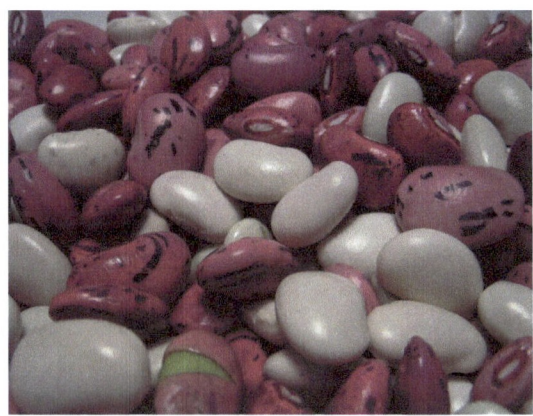

Snacks

Some foods that are usually not considered healthy actually have a low GI.

For example, a Snickers bar is high in calories and fat, but ranks only (41) on the glycemic index.

Other low-GI snacks are milk chocolate (42), Nutella (33), peanuts (13), walnuts (15), corn chips (42), and hummus (6).

High Glycemic Food Examples

Breads

Several types of breads are considered to have a high glycemic index.

After eating high GI breads, blood sugar will rise very quickly.

Breads that have a high glycemic index include white bread, white rolls, baguettes, bagels, black bread and gluten-free bread.

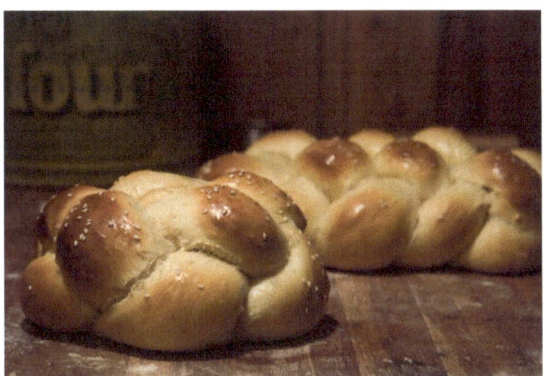

Pasta and Rice

Brown rice pasta has a very high GI.

Other relatively high GI pastas include macaroni and cheese or durum wheat spaghetti.

Some rice has a high glycemic index, including brown rice and jasmine rice.

Rice cakes also have a high GI.

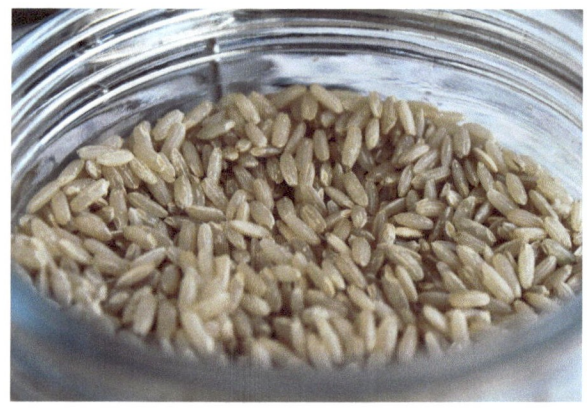

Cereal and Breakfast Foods

Breakfast cereals which are high in carbohydrate levels tend to have the highest GI.

These cereals include: Coco Pops, Cornflakes, Puffed Wheat, Rice Krispies, Weetabix, Golden Grahams and Bran Flakes.

Some cereal grains have a high GI, including barley flakes and millet.

A number of breakfast and bakery products are also included in this category, including doughnuts, croissants and waffles.

Snacks

When it comes to snacks, it's no surprise that many of these fall into the higher GI range.

Pretzels, jelly beans and ice cream are some of the snacks with the highest glycemic index.

Corn chips and soda crackers can be added to that list as well.

Also, any time you add table sugar to a food, the GI increases significantly.

Fruits and Vegetables

Even though we consider fruits and vegetables to be healthy, some have a higher GI than others, including potatoes, parsnips, pineapple and watermelon.

Note that while steamed, mashed, instant and baked potatoes all have a high GI, those that are boiled are actually in the intermediate GI range.

Broad beans are also in this category, though technically they are a legume.

Myth #2:   Fat Makes You Fat.

There is a lot of controversy surrounding fat in our diet. Most of us have been lead to believe that we must eat low fat in order to lose weight and in order to keep our heart healthy.

The problem with this is the same as with carbohydrates, and just assuming that all fat is bad is not going to get us the results we are looking for.

The research on fat and our diets is continuing to change. We are not going to belabor that point in this section, however, I want you to know *that not all fats are created equally.*

There is plenty of evidence that indicates that trans fatty acids are indeed harmful to our bodies. These are the fats that are predominant in many of the processed foods and fast foods that we are exposed to each and every day. **The key** here is to severely limit our intake of highly processed foods and fast foods.

There is more and more evidence mounting to support that fact that we must have a good supply of Omega 3 fatty acids in our diets. These fats are essential to maintaining a healthy hormonal balance in our bodies.

Much of the myth about fat has been perpetuated **due to lack of knowledge** about this particular class of foods. Ask any well intentioned medical practitioner and they are going to preach to you the importance of sticking to the low fat theory because they are convinced that cholesterol is public enemy number 1 when it comes to heart health.

I personally do not subscribe to that notion and I am convinced that cholesterol has very little real impact on heart health.

I feel that this notion has been perpetuated by the pharmaceutical industry and that there is now **a ton of evidence** that indicates that the aggressive use of cholesterol lowering drugs may have deleterious effects instead of all of the benefits that are purported.

Consider this for example: Cholesterol forms part of each and every cell in your body and it is vital to health. It is necessary for maintaining healthy cell walls, making hormones, making vitamin D and for producing bile acids. **Without cholesterol, you will die.**

In addition, **fully half the people with heart disease have perfectly normal cholesterol levels and half the people who have elevated cholesterol levels have perfectly normal hearts without disease.**

There are many clinical studies available now that demonstrate how little difference cholesterol makes in predicting heart disease. One of the classic studies is the **Lyon Diet Heart Study published in the journal Circulation.**

In essence this study looked at 605 patients who had already had a first heart attack and followed them for a four year period between 1988 – 1992. These people had multiple other cardiovascular risk factors including smoking, sedentary lifestyles and high cholesterol.

The results of this study were very interesting because half way through the study the researchers decided to stop because of their startling results.

You see the study included 2 groups. One group was fed a standard "low fat" diet that eliminated fats and cholesterol. The other group was fed a Mediterranean Diet that included lots of olive oil, vegetables and so on.

Want to know what happened?

Half way through the study, the people in the Mediterranean group that included plenty of fats, were noted to be dying at less than half the rate of the "low fat" group. The researchers felt that it was unethical to continue their research protocol and started all of the participants on a Mediterranean diet.

The most interesting thing about this study was that the group that ate the Mediterranean diet, which by the way is way higher in fat than the standard American diet, experienced a nearly ***75% decrease in heart disease*** even though their cholesterol levels did not budge.

Myth #3:   You Must Count Calories to Lose Weight

Calorie counting is ***highly over-rated*** when it comes to weight loss. Don't get me wrong, calories do count but it has been my experience that people who go crazy over counting calories do no better with weight loss than those who do not count calories and in some cases they do worse.

Calorie counting is burdensome and anytime you place too much of a burden on your new eating habits, you will eventually throw your hands up and quit.

If you quit trying to change your eating habits and give up on your weight loss plan entirely, I can assure you that you will not lose weight.

Now with that being said, let's take a look at what calories really mean to us. Calories are indeed a means of tracking but too many people put all of their emphasis on managing their calories. **That does not work.**

It is helpful to understand how many calories your body consumes at rest. This is called your basal metabolic rate (BMR). *The body needs energy from food* (calories) to perform all of its basic functions.

Believe it or not, it **is** possible to eat **too few** calories and this is likely the most important reason to pay attention to your calories. *Eating too few calories can result in your body becoming catabolic and can result in muscle wasting.*

An easy way to estimate your daily calorie needs is to use the following formula.

Women: BMR = 655 + (4.35 x wt in lbs) + (4.7 x Ht in in) – (4.7 x age in yrs)

Men: BMR = 66+ (6.23 x wt in lbs) + (12.7 x Ht in in) – (6.8 x age in yrs)

The old school of nutritional thinking basically teaches that all calories are created equal. Weight loss is based on the calorie in must be less than the calories out equation. ***Nothing could be further from the truth.***

It is important to note that we now know that all fats, carbohydrates and proteins are not created equal. Different fats, carbohydrates and proteins all have different effects on metabolism and our hormonal balance.

The Magic Solution for Weight Loss

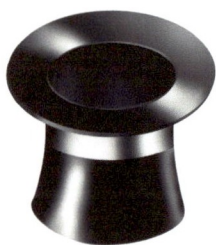

I bet you just jumped straight to this section without looking at anything else. I know. **Everyone** wants that magic solution to make the weight just melt off.

Unfortunately that kind of solution does not exist.

However, this section is about a magic solution that comes as close as anything ever will to making that happen. The magic solution for weight loss is **WATER.**

That's right. Water is essentially a magic solution when it comes to losing weight. I realize that is not what you wanted to hear but the truth is hard to deny.

Hold on. Don't toss the book aside just yet. After all, you are here to learn how to shed those unwanted pounds. Aren't you?

Most people do not drink nearly enough water to support their daily metabolic needs. In fact, we are so inundated by flavored drinks, juices and sodas, that most people drink little or no pure water at all.

If you are not drinking enough water to keep your body hydrated, your weight loss battle quickly moves from being a small fight to becoming a very large battle.

Here are a few of the reasons why water is so important:

- Water is essential to helping your body eliminate stored fat. In order to remove fat form your system, you really need your liver in top shape. When it is deprived of the water it needs, your metabolic machinery does not function properly and you essentially create a backlog of metabolic waste that slows the entire system down. ***Water is essential to your liver's ability to effectively metabolize stored fat.***

- Water is also essential to maintaining optimal kidney function. As you metabolize the fat stores in your body, you create a mess of toxins and waste byproducts. In order to flush these waste substances from your system you need a healthy filtering system. ***If you are not keeping your body hydrated, your kidneys are unable to effectively remove the waste from your body and again fat metabolism will slow down.***

- Water is a natural **diuretic.** During the course of a day, most of us will retain some degree of fluid. These fluid shifts are aggravated by our sedentary life styles, medications we might be taking, our salt intake, hormonal imbalances and more importantly our state of hydration. If you are going to be able to remove this fluid buildup and stop fluid retention, you have to drink plenty of water. Water is likely the best diuretic we have at our disposal. It amazes me how many people think just the opposite. I hear this all the time. I have cut back on my water intake because I am holding fluid. ***Unless you have a failing heart or a failing renal (kidney) system, nothing could be further from the truth.***

- Water is a great laxative. Your bowels depend on a good supply of water to keep things moving. When you do not get enough weater in your system, you colon is forced to try to salvage every drop that it can before waste is eliminated. This will often times result in constipation. ***If you want your bowels to work, make sure that you are getting plenty of water into the pipeline***.

When we talk about water there is a number of suggestions about how much water you should be drinking. Most people are familiar with the fact that they should be drinking 8 to 10 glasses a day; that is 60 to 80 ounces. This is a good estimate for many people but if you are overweight that might not be enough.

In order to better estimate the amount of water you need, I suggest the following formula. ***You should be drinking at least half your body weight in ounces of water each and every day:*** more than that; if you are active and sweating throughout the day.

For example, if you weigh 200 pounds then you should be drinking at least 100 ounces of water just to ***maintain your basic state of hydration***. I know, that seems like a lot and I can hear you moaning right now saying if I drink all of that I will never get out of the bathroom.

However, ***if you are serious about losing weight and improving your health, you are going to have to get busy taking care of yourself***.

Your body is by far the most precious asset you have on this earth. ***Do not continue to abuse it or it will eventually fail on*** *you*. When your body fails, you will no longer be able to take care of all of those other people in your life that need you around to care for them.

Many people mistake thirst for hunger. Therefore, when you begin to feel hungry, make sure that you stop and drink at least 8 ounces of water first. Give yourself about 20 minutes and then if you are still hungry, go ahead and eat.

The Hormonal Connection to Weight Loss

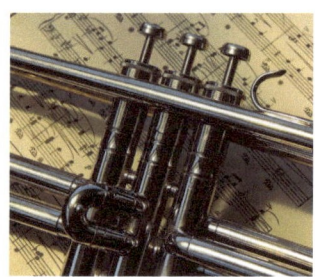

Every one of us has heard about hormones. They control ***every metabolic action that goes on in our bodies.*** When it comes to weight gain we all tend to think of thyroid hormones and insulin. Although these are 2 very important hormones in regards to weight loss and energy metabolism, there are several that we need to discuss in this section.

This book is really not about hormones. That subject is way too dense to tackle in the context of what we are trying to accomplish here. However, I think it is important that you at least have an idea of how the hormonal systems affect you when it comes to losing weight.

This area of weight loss is often overlooked and leads to an immense amount of frustration for would be dieters.

Have you ever failed at losing weight despite a wholehearted effort to diet?

Have you gained weight even though you stuck to your plan religiously?

If you have experienced the frustration of doing everything you were asked to do but nonetheless continued to gain weight, you might have a hormonal imbalance that is hindering your progress.

The Key Players in the Hormonal Symphony

When it comes to a discussion of hormones there are several key players that we need to discuss. When I am discussing hormonal imbalance with my patients in the clinic, I like to use the analogy of a symphony.

All of us have heard wonderful music being played by a symphony orchestra at one time or another. When all of those players are working together in perfect harmony, in tune with each other; they make beautiful music.

If one or more of them begin to play off beat or get out of tune the music is less than desirable. This is what happens in or bodies as well. We go along year after year with all of our systems in perfect harmony, then for some reason we seem to begin to lose our edge. *We get out of sync and we often don't know why.*

As we age, all of us are **constantly changing**. The foods we eat, the activity we perform, the jobs we do, the problems we have with other people, our stress levels, our sleep patterns all have an impact on how overall wellbeing.

Unfortunately, it is not until we "**fall apart**" that we begin to pay attention to all of these subtle changes.

These changes are related to a host of factors and our hormonal balance is one of the primary factors.

Here are some of the key hormones and how they interact within us.

Insulin:

Insulin is a major factor in the weight loss puzzle. Our diets are usually filled with highly processed foods and way too much sugar. As we go about our business from year to year, insulin accumulates and gets higher and higher in our system. Insulin as we discussed earlier is responsible for transporting glucose to the cells that need it for energy. As the levels increase over time, we tend to store more and more of that sugar in our liver where it is converted to fat. *The higher our insulin levels, the better and more efficient we are at storing fat instead of burning fat.*

Thyroid hormones:

The thyroid gland is a major controller of metabolism and energy. As we age we tend to see a decline in normal thyroid function. As the thyroid gland declines in its ability to produce thyroid hormones, we tend to gain weight and we tend to have more fatigue. Most of us when dealing with fatigue find ourselves slowing down. *The less active we are the more we hold onto excess calories and the more weight we tend to gain.*

Cortisol:

Cortisol is a stress hormone in our bodies. The more stress we deal with on a daily basis the more we activate the adrenal system and the more cortisol we produce. One of the untoward effects of excess cortisol is weight gain. In discussing this issue with many patients, *most people do not realize how much of a negative impact that cortisol has on our system.* Disruptions in our normal sleep pattern, too much stress in our lives, and poor nutrition activate the adrenal system and excess cortisol is the result.

Leptin:

Leptin is another hormone that is being talked about a lot in respect to weight gain these days. ***Anytime you go on a diet and reduce your calorie intake, leptin levels fall and fat burning is dramatically reduced.*** Leptin's main function is to protect your body against starvation and when you restrict calories too severely during a diet, you trigger this system to hang onto your fat stores. Your body views these fat stores as your biggest asset to prevent you from staving.

This list includes only a few of the major hormones that affect your ability to lose weight. As you can see this topic can be quite extensive and if you feel like you are dealing with a hormonal imbalance, you need to discuss that with your primary care physician or another physician that is education in helping you restore your hormonal balance.

Alcohol and Artificial Sweeteners

No discussion on weight loss would be complete without some attention to the topics of alcohol and artificial sweeteners. I have saved this section for last because you are not going to enjoy what I have to say about either of these.

When it comes to weight loss, some things that are considered acceptable, nutritional practices, ***do not work.***

Alcohol:

In regards to alcohol, it ***is important to remember that alcohol is detrimental to your weight loss efforts.*** You may have been told that some forms of alcohol, red wines in particular, may be beneficial for heart health. Although I believe that to be true, alcohol in any form is likely ***detrimental to your weight loss efforts.***

Alcohol is considered a **carbohydrate**, but your body processes it differently from other carbohydrates. The body treats alcohol as a **toxin** and therefore attempts to process alcohol calories before all other calories in an attempt to clear the toxins from the bloodstream.

As other calories wait in line to be processed the body senses an increase in calories and stores some of the excess calories away in the fat cells. Not what we want to be doing when we are trying to lose weight.

In short, it is prudent to ***avoid alcohol when you are trying to lose weight.***

Artificial Sweeteners:

Most weight loss programs allow, and some encourage, artificial sweeteners. I do not.

The main issue with artificial sweeteners is that ***the brain cannot tell the difference between artificial sweeteners and sugar***. Although there are typically no calories in the artificial sweeteners, they stimulate an insulin response just like sugar.

If you recall from our earlier discussion that insulin, at higher levels, is primarily a fat storing hormone and we do not need it stimulated by an artificial sweetener.

Artificial sweeteners also signal your taste buds that the sweet stuff has arrived. This gets translated by the brain that nutrition has arrived and when the artificial sweetener reaches the small intestine and there is no nutrition, it creates confusion in the system that essentially triggers you to keep eating. ***This often leads to over eating.***

Almost every diet or sugar-free product on the market today has some type of artificial sweetener added to it. ***Read ingredient labels very carefully.***

If you need a more natural alternative to sugar and artificial sweeteners, I would recommend that you try **Stevia**. Stevia offers a wonderful natural alternative to both sugar and artificial sweeteners. Stevia is derived form an herb and is almost free of calories. ***Unlike artificial sweeteners it is not considered to be toxic to the body and provides a great tasting alternative***.

The Simply Weight Loss Plan

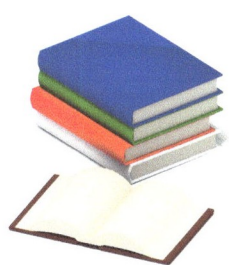

Our simply weight loss plan is based on ***sound nutrition and education***. As you can tell by now, I believe that the only way to truly control your destiny is to take control of your life as a whole. That means that you have to educate yourself about how things in your life truly affect you. Weight loss is no different.

If you want to be successful at playing the weight loss game, you must be educated.

- You need to make sure that you have a good understanding of how carbohydrates, fats and proteins are working in your body.

- You have to be able to recognize which foods you are eating are helping you win the game and which ones are slowing down your progress.

Once you have mastered these concepts then you are ready to put it all into practice.

Our approach is really quite simple to grasp and even easier to stick with. I found out many years ago that the best way to create success was to break down your project into small easily managed steps that anyone could understand.

Once you have got that, your **primary job** is to learn how to master those steps and integrate them into your life with such regularity that they become a part of your everyday experience.

Weight loss is like any other task you are trying to master. *If you do not practice the task until it has become second nature,* you will ultimately slip right back into your old routines and when you do you will go right back to where you started.

Albert Einstein once said, "Insanity is doing the same thing over and over while expecting different results."

The same is true here.

If you can make the changes we have discussed and continue to monitor and track until you do these things naturally, you will have success. *If you are unwilling to make the necessary changes, then you will FAIL.*

You cannot keep practicing bad habits and never expect to get bad results. That kind of thinking does not work and is only appropriate for people who are lying to themselves.

In order to keep this process as simple as possible, I am going to jump right into the program. As we go we will have to add some additional information. Things are always changing and we will provide those updates as we go.

Before we start, I would like to *encourage you to make sure that you discuss any weight loss program with your primary care physician.* Just in case he/she has any concerns that might affect your health.

Personally, I can't imagine any medical problem in existence that will not improve by taking these actions. In fact, there is a plethora of information on the subject. If you are overweight and your health is less than optimal, cleaning up your diet and losing weight can only make you feel better. ***Feeling better will improve your outlook on life and when we feel better we respond better to everything in life.***

That being said, let's get started.

Phase 1 – Elimination

As we go through this lesson, I will try to make things as simple and understandable as possible. In doing that, realize that some of the concepts we are discussing are much more complex than I portray them.

The idea here is to help you understand how to get started in your weight loss quest. As we go, it will be up to you to keep learning. The better you understand what is happening inside your body the better your food choices will become and the more success you will experience.

As we begin to use this program there are 6 basic food groups that I am going to have you eliminate from your diet. Notice that I said **ELIMINATE**. I didn't say reduce, cut back on or slow down. I said **ELIMINATE**. That means that to start I don't want these things to pass between your lips.

We need to eliminate:

1.   **Sugar** -   Notice that I did not say carbohydrates. I said sugar. This means that we are to eliminate all processed sugars. More on this later.

2.   **Bread** -   This includes all forms of bread including wheat.

3.   **Rice** -   This includes all rice even brown rice.

4.   **Pasta** -   This includes all types of past including wheat and whole grain.

5.   **Potatoes**   This includes all potatoes including sweet potatoes.

6.   **Fast Food**   This includes all fast food. If you can get it from a drive thru it needs to be eliminated for now.

I know, I can hear all of the moaning already. Before you decide to quit before you get started make sure you keep reading as I will try to explain what we are doing and why. Once you understand that this is a ***very temporary situation, it will make it much more palatable.***

As you can see I am asking you to eliminate all of these highly processed foods.

There is a really good reason for this. In fact, there are several really good reasons. We know without a doubt that highly processed foods contain a ton of sugar and bad fats. Remember some of the discussions earlier about trans fats? Well this is why we need to get rid of all of these foods for now.

The processed foods listed above increase the insulin levels in your body. As we increase insulin, we basically become more effective at storing fat than we do at burning fat. In a nutshell, that means that even if you eat the same number of calories every day, as you increase insulin levels you are not able to burn those calories as effectively and you will store more fat as a result.

Not only that but these foods ***are known to increase inflammation in our body and we know that inflammation wreaks havoc all through our bodies.*** Inflammation increases our risk of heart disease, joint pains, join stiffness, weight gain, aging and a host of other issues that none of us really want or need to be dealing with.

The main reason we want to eliminate these foods, is to give our bodies a fighting chance at reducing some of the insulin that is present. As insulin levels decline in our bodies we naturally become more efficient at burning fat and that is exactly what we need to be doing. **Burn fat burn**!

Now just so you are not freaking out, you only need to go through this elimination phase for the first 2 to 4 weeks of the program. That is sufficient time to start your weight loss and reset yourself metabolically.

Once we know we are able to start shedding the pounds and burn the fat, we can think about adding back in some of these foods. However, I do not recommend that you eat anything from these classes of foods more often than 2 or 3 times a week: **Period.** They are just too inflammatory in nature and many of them will eventually wreck your progress if you are not careful.

Phase 2 – Tracking Your Weight

Here is where I often times get some derogatory comments on my program. There is a host of opinions about whether you should weigh or not. I personally think it is beneficial to weigh each and every day and I will explain why in just a moment.

I do have one rule about daily weighs, however, that I must convey right now. If you step on the scales and you feel "bad" or "negative", you need to ***put your scales away and only weigh on a weekly basis***. If you can use your scales as a constructive devise to help you learn what is happening in your body, then daily weighs may be beneficial.

I am convinced that much of the problem we have with weight is not because the foods we eat are all bad for us. In fact, some of the studies that have been done in regards to food sensitivities seem to suggest that all of might have a handful of very specific foods that affect us in a very negative way.

When you eat a food that your gastrointestinal track is sensitive to, you will notice that you often times feel full, bloated, you will have increased gas and belching and you will often feel very tired. ***That is your bodies way of telling you that what you just did does not work.***

I believe that we can use our daily weigh-ins to help us identify some of the foods that wreck our weight loss program. This is why I like to see you weigh daily.

If you are stepping on your scales each and every day at the same time of day, you can see the small 1, 2 and 3 pound weight changes that will occur.

By monitoring these changes and correlating that to your tracking (the phase 3 component of our program) you will be able to eliminate some of these highly inflammatory foods.

The reason this is essential to do is that none of us are exactly the same and just because a particular food does not work for me does not mean that it will not work for you. The only way to know for sure is to track and monitor and pay attention to the details of your weight loss plan.

If you are one of those people that cannot tolerate daily weighs then you should *at least monitor your weight on a weekly basis* to make sure that you are keeping yourself on track.

Study after study suggests that those who weigh themselves more frequently are more successful at losing and maintaining their weight loss.

The National Weight Control Registry, a database of members who have lost an average of 66 pounds and kept the weight off for nearly 6 years, shows one positive habit – *75% of those in the Registry weigh themselves at least one time each week*.

And the participants who **weighed themselves daily** did even better over the long term. I recommend you weigh yourself daily. This way you will "**catch**" when your weight starts to go up or is not moving.

Make sure you weigh yourself at the same time every day to establish a ritual… the best time is in the morning right after you wake up and go to the bathroom.

Then chart this in your journal next to your food entries or picture library.

Remember *that you will have normal daily fluctuations* and also that the scale does not register the ratio between muscle and fat. For this you can get a body fat scale or use a tape measure once a week to check your waist and thigh area.

The main thing is to create these rituals… *this is what people who lose weight permanently do, so you might benefit as well.*

As we will discuss next, tracking is the essential key to long term success.

Phase 3 – Tracking Your Progress

If you want to be a success in any aspect of life, it is essential that *you track, track, and track some more.* If you are not tracking your results then you will never really understand what works and what does not. When it comes to weight loss this will be your definite demise.

Tracking your food intake is essential to long term success.

- **First**, you need to be able to monitor your caloric intake. As you already know, I am not a big fan of meticulous calorie counting. I prefer to use estimations but it is nice to be able to glance at your tracking sheet and know that we are in the ball park.

- **Secondly**, if you are not tracking and writing down everything you eat, you will never be able to identify any of the problem foods that are causing the yo-yo rollercoaster you have been living with all of these years.

That being said, you have to track you food intake. It doesn't matter how you do this as long as you are doing it. I prefer to track a week at a time on a sheet of paper (I have included a copy of my personal favorite tracking sheet in the appendix). If you are a technology person, there are a number of tracking programs available to your computer and smart phone.

The key to tracking success is to make sure that you are using a method that allows you to keep good records. You will need to make sure that you include everything that goes into your mouth on your tracking list. This includes your regular meals, what you are drinking and snacks you might have. It also needs to include those small bites of whatever seems to just jump into your mouth throughout the day. We like to ignore those things but they all count.

Keeping a food diary *can double a person's weight loss*, according to a study from Kaiser Permanente's Center for Health Research**. The findings, from one of the largest and longest running weight loss maintenance trials ever conducted, are something to take seriously.

"The more food records people kept, the more weight they lost," said lead author Jack Hollis Ph.D., a researcher at Kaiser Permanente's Center for Health Research in Portland, Oregon. "Those who kept daily food records lost twice as much weight as those who kept no records. It seems that the simple act of writing down what you eat encourages people to consume fewer calories."

"Keeping a food diary doesn't have to be a formal thing. Just the act of scribbling down what you eat on a Post-It note, sending yourself e-mails tallying each meal, or sending yourself a text message will suffice.

It's the process of reflecting on what you eat that helps us become aware of our habits, and hopefully change our behavior," says Keith Bachman, MD, a Weight Management Initiative member.

And now that most phones have cameras, I have found that taking pictures of every meal and then uploading them daily to be highly effective.

Putting It All Together

"You must begin to think of yourself as becoming the person you want to be"- David Viscott

So there you go, you have the first 3 phases.

Now we need to get to work. Before we do though I know what you are thinking. "What am I going to eat?" I asked you to eliminate 6 food groups from your diet and guess what, you don't seem to have much left. If that is where you are at, then I can tell you without a doubt that ***you need this program***.

When I get this question in my clinic I always answer the same way. ***You can eat anything that is not on the phase 1 elimination list***. That leaves a ton of vegetables, lots of lean meats and eggs, and fruits. In addition, you should be drinking a ton of **water.**

I recommend that you drink half your body weight in ounces of water every day. That is, if you weigh 200 pounds then you should be drinking 100 ounces of water each day just to maintain your hydration state.

Your body was designed to eat a meal every 3 to 4 hours. I refer to this as a **metabolic cycle**. That is, when you put food into the system, your body will break down the food, absorb the nutrients, elevate blood sugar and insulin levels and realize that it is hungry again in about 3 to 4 hours. If you are going to optimize your metabolism, you will need to cater to this system. It will not adjust to you just because of your work schedule.

If you eat your meals too close together your **blood sugar will be elevated throughout the day and you are more likely to store fat than to burn it**. If you eat your meals too far apart, you might enter a catabolic (muscle wasting) state.

Here are a few more guidelines that I suggest you consider as you put your plan into action.

- Always try to get your first meal of the day **within 1 hour of waking up**. If this is a challenge to you, drinking a protein shake when you first get up in the morning is an easy fix.

- Try to eat any complex **carbohydrates and fruits early in the day.** This will ensure that your insulin sensitivity is high so that the carbs can be used for energy, growth and repair.

- Try to get some type of lean protein and hour or two **prior to going to bed**. This will provide your muscles with a steady stream of amino acids and prevent your body from going into a catabolic (muscle wasting) state.

- **Never eat your carbohydrates by themselves**. It is best to combine these with some form of protein. This will keep the carbs from spiking your blood sugar and insulin levels. When insulin spikes it creates a fat storing environment in our bodies.

- **Eat the right type of fats**. Be sure to keep plenty of Omega 3 fatty acids in your diet. I recommend at least 2 to 4 grams each day. Healthy fats are essential for weight loss and hormonal balance. Try to eat fish at least 3 times each week.

- **Eat the right carbohydrates**. Vegetables are by far your best source of carbohydrates. Avoid processed sugars as they spike insulin and result in increased fat storage. You should also work hard to get **at least 25 to 30 grams of fiber into your diet each and every day.**

Fruits are acceptable. I am a fan of all fruits. However, when you are trying to lose weight I would encourage you to **limit your fruit intake to 2 servings a day**. Remember that a serving of most fruits is about the size of a tennis ball. Also note that some fruits seem to slow fat loss. My favorite fruits are apples, oranges, grapefruits, and berries.

I encourage you to use spices of all kinds, but use these "super spices" every day if you can: Basil, Cardamom, Cayenne, Cilantro, Cinnamon, Ginger, Parsley, and Turmeric. (Curry can be a great source of several of these spices, so feel free to add it to your vegetable soups or meat dishes for added health and weight loss benefits!)

These spices are very important as they will help **increase adiponectin and help balance blood sugar.**

Avoid all artificial sweeteners. The research is becoming clear: artificial sweeteners like aspartame (Nutrasweet) and Splenda mimic the same insulin response as natural sugars, not to mention other side-effects and potential harm to your brain.

Don't drink your calories. No fruit juices, sodas, etc... This is a fast way to weight gain! Some people **literally lose up to 10 pounds in the first few weeks of their new diet simply by giving up soda alone.** Remember, diet sodas contain artificial sweeteners so stay away from both regular and diet!

Create a cheat meal once each week. There is a ton of evidence that supports the use of a cheat meal for several reasons. First, just knowing that you can cheat seems to help alleviate some of the psychological stress that hinders our progress. Secondly, there is evidence to support that including a cheat meal might prevent the plateau effect that we often see with weight loss.

I look at this sort of like I do interval exercise training. If you *keep your body confused metabolically it might prevent the plateaus we often see with weight loss programs.*

Cheat Meal Suggestions

Here are a few suggestions that I have found that work better in most cases than more "controlled" approaches placing restrictions on what foods may or may not be eaten.

Suggestion #1   Let Go of the Guilt

This is the ***most important guideline*** of the Cheat Meal.

Take a leap of faith and go for it; trust me, it works.

When you understand how the body works, you understand that strategic cheating is ultimately what is going to propel your results and progress to a whole new level.

There is nothing to feel guilty about. Eat as you please and don't think twice about "limiting" what you can and can't eat.

Suggestion #2   Avoid Overeating and Stuffing Yourself

Although I truly want you to eat the foods you crave without remorse, ***I do NOT want you to gorge yourself.***

When you are eating, it is important to realize that there is ***a disconnect between your stomach and your brain.*** That's right. It takes about 20 minutes after your stomach is full for your brain to "get the message". In order to avoid overeating and gorging you have to be aware of how much you have eaten.

Eat until you are moderately full ***(don't stuff yourself)***, and then wait until you are at least moderately hungry again before tackling your next craving.

The Cheat Day is not meant to be a "**binge**"; it's meant to be an enjoyable psychological and physiological outlet to hasten results and increase dietary adherence. Don't abuse it.

Suggestion #3   Don't Skip Meals

While you may be looking forward to a big buffet or have an evening event planned, I don't want you to "save" your appetite for a "main event" so to speak.

Your body is designed to be fed every 3 to 4 hours. ***Do not deprive your system so that you can over eat later.***

Studies have shown that prolonged periods of overfeeding or "cheating" are needed in order to elicit a substantial leptin response and bring your body back into ***"fat burning mode".***

Make a day—not a meal—out of it.

Suggestion #4   Avoid Excess Alcohol Consumption

A beer or two or a glass of wine is fine, but overdoing it with the alcohol intake on   your Cheat Day can have significant negative effects.

Studies have shown that excess alcohol consumption has an immediate negative impact on leptin levels, which essentially cancels out everything we are trying to accomplish with the Cheat Day.

In all honesty, I prefer that alcohol is avoided as it's an area where many people push the envelope, but I'd be lying if I told you that I didn't regular enjoy a glass or two of red wine on my Cheat Day.

This day is all about enjoyment. Eat the foods you love, don't feel guilty, speed along your fat loss, and reap the many psychological and physiological benefits of taking some "time off" from the regular program. ***This is YOUR day.***

Appendix

Weight Loss Tracking Sheet

DATE: ___/___/2012	DATE: ___/___/2012	DATE: ___/___/2012	DATE: ___/___/2012	DATE: ___/___/2012	DATE: ___/___/2012	DATE: ___/___/2012
WEIGHT _____ LBS	WEIGHT _____ LBS	WEIGHT _____ LBS	WEIGHT _____ LBS	WEIGHT _____ LBS	WEIGHT _____ LBS	WEIGHT _____ LBS
BREAKFAST	BREAKFAST	BREAKFAST	BREAKFAST	BREAKFAST	BREAKFAST	BREAKFAST
LUNCH	LUNCH	LUNCH	LUNCH	LUNCH	LUNCH	LUNCH
SUPPER	SUPPER	SUPPER	SUPPER	SUPPER	SUPPER	SUPPER
SNACKS AND FREE FOODS	SNACKS AND FREE FOODS	SNACKS AND FREE FOODS	SNACKS AND FREE FOODS	SNACKS AND FREE FOODS	SNACKS AND FREE FOODS	SNACKS AND FREE FOODS
PROBLEMS & MISTAKES	PROBLEMS & MISTAKES	PROBLEMS & MISTAKES	PROBLEMS & MISTAKES	PROBLEMS & MISTAKES	PROBLEMS & MISTAKES	PROBLEMS & MISTAKES
EXERCISE	EXERCISE	EXERCISE	EXERCISE	EXERCISE	EXERCISE	EXERCISE

About the Author

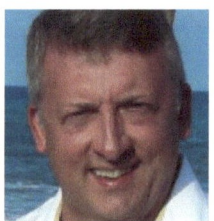

Dr. Mike Cockrell is a practicing family physician in Senatobia, Mississippi. Dr. Cockrell completed his undergraduate education in Medical Technology at the University of Mississippi in 1984. After working in this field for a number of years, Dr. Cockrell returned to complete his Doctorate of Medicine (MD) at the University of Tennessee in Memphis, TN.

After completing his residency training at the University of Tennessee / Baptist Memorial Hospital – Tipton program in 2002, Dr. Cockrell established Cockrell Family Medical Center, PC in Senatobia, MS where he is currently in private practice.

Dr. Cockrell is Board Certified in Family Practice by the American Board of Family Practice and is certified in Age Management Medicine by the Cenegenics Education and Research Foundation. Dr. Cockrell's primary interest is in the area of prevention and he has a particular interest in hormonal optimization and the effects of hormone imbalance on weight gain.

In addition to managing a full clinical practice, Dr. Cockrell is also co-owner of several other businesses and he considers himself an entrepreneur at heart. Dr. Cockrell is actively involved in teaching and training small business owners and individuals how to enhance their offline and online presence using a host of tools available both offline and online. He is an active blogger and enjoys reading, writing and travelling. He is also an avid art and coin collector.

Additional Resources:

http://www.DoctorCockrell.com

http://www.DrMikeCockrell.com

http://www.CockrellCoins.net

http://www.facebook.com/CockrellFamilyMedical

http://www.facebook.com/LaurelRosePublishing